I0697371

PROSTATE HEALTH REVOLUTION:

Empowering Men to Take Control of Their Well-Being

Amber H. Austin

TABLE OF CONTENTS

All rights reserved. No part of this publication may be reproduced, distributed, or transmitted in any form or by any means, including photocopying, recording, or other electronic or mechanical methods, without the prior written permission of the publisher, except in the case of brief quotations embodied in critical reviews and certain other noncommercial uses permitted by copyright law.

Copyright © **AMBER H. AUSTIN,** 2023.

INTRODUCTION

We invite you to join us in the Prostate Health Revolution as we set out on a mission to enable men all around the world to take charge of their health. It can be simple to disregard our health in today's hectic and demanding environment, especially when it comes to delicate issues like prostate health. The time has come for us to overcome these obstacles, nevertheless, and adopt a proactive attitude toward our general well-being.

The production of seminal fluid and the maintenance of normal sexual function are both tasks performed by the prostate gland, an essential component of the male reproductive system. Many men are not aware of the various problems that their prostate health may encounter, even though they should be.

Prostatitis, benign prostatic hyperplasia (BPH), and prostate cancer are among the conditions that can significantly lower a man's quality of life.

It's time to revolutionize the way we think about prostate health. We shouldn't just sit back and wait for symptoms to appear, nor should we only follow the advice of doctors. Instead, we must arm ourselves with the information, comprehension, and tools needed to take charge of our health.

We will explore the numerous facets of prostate health in this book, including the most frequent ailments, risk factors, safeguards, and possible treatments. We'll also throw some light on the psychological effects that these ailments may have, enabling men to address their worries and fears and get the help they require.

We intend to give you, the reader, a thorough manual that goes beyond merely providing information. We want to spark a fire within you that will inspire you to put your prostate health first and make healthy adjustments in all facets of your life. The information in this book will act as a road map for you as you attempt to negotiate the frequently difficult terrain of prostate health.

The Prostate Health Revolution is here to empower you, whether you are a young man looking for preventive measures or an older man coping with prostate-related diseases. Together, we will dismantle the stigmas associated with prostate health, combat societal taboos, and create a welcoming environment where men may freely express their worries and seek advice.

Are you prepared to assume responsibility for your health? Join this revolution with us, and let's empower guys all around the world to put their prostate health first and live their lives to the fullest.

CHAPTER 1. UNDERSTANDING OF PROSTATE HEALTH

A little gland called the prostate, which is part of the male reproductive system is extremely important to reproductive health.

The urethra, the tube that takes urine and sperm out of the body, is surrounded by the prostate gland, which is a component of the male reproductive system and is situated right below the bladder. It is a tiny gland, about the size of a walnut, made up of both muscle and glandular tissue. The prostate gland performs several different bodily tasks.

The synthesis and secretion of seminal fluid is one of the prostate gland's primary tasks. Semen, the fluid that carries and feeds sperm after ejaculation, contains seminal fluid, which is a vital component.

Semen is created when a secretion from the prostate's glandular tissue interacts with sperm and fluids from other reproductive organs. The sperm are fed and shielded by this fluid, which improves their survival and mobility.

The seminal fluid is propelled during ejaculation by the smooth muscles within the prostate gland. To drive the semen into the urethra and out of the body, these muscles tighten in unison. Additionally, the prostate gland has valves that keep urine and seminal fluid separate during ejaculation.

The prostate gland is important in terms of fertility. The sperm can thrive and travel through the female reproductive system to reach the egg for fertilization in the seminal fluid that the prostate produces.

Additionally, several proteins and enzymes that are produced by the prostate gland help activate and improve sperm motility, enhancing the likelihood of successful fertilization. Therefore, good sperm production and fertility depend on the prostate gland operating properly.

1.1: How The Prostate Changes Over Time

In men, the prostate is a tiny gland the size of a walnut that is situated below the bladder. By creating a fluid that feeds and carries sperm, it performs a critical part of the reproductive system. The prostate experiences several changes over time that are impacted by aging, hormonal changes, and additional variables like heredity and lifestyle.

The term "benign prostatic hyperplasia" (BPH) refers to one of the most prevalent prostate alterations associated with aging. Prostate enlargement, often known as BPH, primarily affects males over the age of 50. Dihydrotestosterone (DHT) and estrogen levels in particular rise as men age, altering the body's hormonal equilibrium. These hormonal changes cause prostate cells to multiply, which causes the gland to expand.

Weak urine flow, more frequent urination, and trouble emptying the bladder are all urinary symptoms of BPH.

An elevated risk of contracting prostate cancer is another key change that might take place in the prostate over time. The most prevalent type of cancer in males is prostate cancer, and the risk of developing it rises with age. Although the precise causes of prostate cancer are not entirely understood, several factors can affect risk, including race (men of African-American descent are at increased risk) and specific genetic abnormalities. For early detection and successful management of prostate cancer, routine PSA screening and monitoring are crucial.

Prostatitis, an infection that causes the prostate gland to become inflamed, may also affect the prostate.
Although bacterial infections can induce prostatitis, the precise cause isn't always recognized. It may cause symptoms like pelvic pain or discomfort, urination problems, and sexual dysfunction. Alpha-blockers or anti-inflammatory drugs are frequently used as

additional treatments for non-bacterial prostatitis in addition to antibiotics for bacterial prostatitis.

Finally, aging-related hormonal changes can also have an impact on the prostate. The main male sex hormone testosterone gradually declines with age, and this decline can result in a variety of alterations in prostate structure and function. However, more research is still needed to determine the precise connection between hormone levels and prostate health.

In conclusion, the prostate experiences several changes as it ages. An enlarged prostate known as benign prostatic hyperplasia (BPH), which is common in older men, can cause symptoms related to the urinary system. With advancing age, the risk of acquiring prostate cancer also rises, calling for ongoing surveillance. People of any age can get prostatitis or prostate gland irritation. As one age, maintaining optimal prostate health can be achieved by being aware of these changes and receiving proper medical care as necessary.

CHAPTER 2: COMMON PROSTATE CONDITIONS

As a person ages, the prostate, a tiny gland in men that is situated behind the bladder, alters in several ways. Both typical aging-related changes and specific disorders that may affect the prostate fall under the category of these alterations. Let's examine both points in depth.

Normal age-related changes

Benign prostate enlargement (BPH) BPH, or benign prostatic hyperplasia, is a non-cancerous disorder in which the prostate gland steadily enlarges with advancing age. Urinary symptoms include frequent urination, poor urine flow, difficulty starting or stopping urination, and the sensation of incomplete emptying may result from the pressure the expanding prostate may put on the urethra.

Reduced Prostate Secretions

Age may cause a reduction in prostatic fluid output. This might alter the consistency of semen and have an impact on fertility.

Specific Conditions that can affect the prostate

2.1: Benign Prostatic Hyperplasia (BPH)

Symptoms

BPH is characterized by urinary symptoms and is brought on by an enlarged prostate gland. Frequent urination, weak urine flow, difficulty starting and stopping urination, dribbling after urination, and the sensation that the bladder has not completely emptied are all possible symptoms.

Risk factors

Hormonal changes are thought to have a part in the risk of BPH, which rises with age. Family history, obesity, and certain illnesses including diabetes and heart disease are additional risk factors.

Diagnosis

A digital rectal exam (DRE) and assessment of the patient's medical history are frequently carried out. Other examinations could involve ultrasonography, a urine flow study, and a blood test for prostate-specific antigen (PSA).

Treatment options

Depending on the severity of the symptoms, BPH treatment options may include watchful waiting, dietary changes, 5-alpha-reductase inhibitors or alpha-blockers, transurethral microwave therapy or laser therapy, or surgery (prostatectomy or transurethral resection of the prostate).

2.2: Prostatitis

Prostatitis, an inflammation of the prostate gland, can result in urine symptoms, pelvic pain, discomfort during ejaculation, and occasionally flu-like symptoms. Acute bacterial prostatitis, persistent bacterial prostatitis, chronic prostatitis/chronic pelvic pain syndrome (CPPS), and silent inflammatory prostatitis are among the various kinds of prostatitis.

Risk factors

Depending on the kind, risk factors for prostatitis may include a history of urinary tract infections, past bouts of prostatitis, a recent bladder infection, or catheter use, and certain sexual behaviors.

Diagnosis

A medical history evaluation, physical examination (including a DRE), study of the urine and prostate fluid, and occasionally imaging studies or cystoscopy are required for the diagnosis.

Prostatitis treatment options

Depending on the type, treatment for prostatitis may entail prostate massage, anti-inflammatory drugs, painkillers, pain management, and lifestyle changes.

2.3: Prostate Cancer

The worry of getting prostate cancer is one of the most prevalent worries among men. Even though prostate cancer is a terrible condition, it's vital to understand that the majority of men who are diagnosed with the disease do not pass away from it. Numerous individuals with prostate cancer in the early stages can receive successful treatment and go on to lead long healthy lives.

The discomfort or shame connected with prostate tests is another major worry. It's crucial to keep in mind that prostate exams and screenings are a regular component of men's healthcare and are not something to feel embarrassed about. Anxiety before these exams can be reduced by being upfront and honest with your healthcare professional about any worries or queries you may have.

Symptoms

Prostate cancer in its early stages may not show any symptoms at all. As the condition worsens, symptoms could include weight loss that isn't explained, erectile dysfunction, urinary issues (such as frequent urination, poor urine flow, or blood in the pee), and hip, back, or pelvic pain.

Risk factors

Age (prostate cancer is more common in older men), family history, race (men of African descent are at higher risk), and specific genetic variants are risk factors for prostate cancer.

Diagnosis

A DRE, blood tests (including PSA levels), imaging tests (such as ultrasound, MRI, or bone scan), and a prostate biopsy are frequently combined to make the diagnosis.

Treatment options

Prostate cancer treatments vary depending on the cancer's stage, general health, and patient preferences. Active surveillance (monitoring without immediate therapy), surgery, chemotherapy, immunotherapy, radiation therapy, hormone therapy, or targeted therapy.

2.4: Prostatic Abscess

Pus builds up inside the prostate gland, causing a prostatic abscess, a rare but deadly ailment. The reproductive system heavily depends on the prostate gland, a little organ in men that is situated below the bladder. It creates a fluid to feed and cover the sperm.

When the prostate gland becomes infected, prostatic abscesses may form. Bacteria, which can spread from other regions of the body or enter the prostate through the urethra, are the most frequent cause of infection. Urinary tract infections, prostate hypertrophy, and particular medical operations involving the prostate are additional causes of prostatic abscesses.

Symptoms

Depending on how severe the infection is, a prostatic abscess can present with a variety of symptoms. Common signs and symptoms include lower back or abdomen discomfort, frequent or difficult urination, blood in the urine, fever, chills, and an overall feeling of being unwell. In some circumstances, the abscess may rupture, allowing the infection to spread to more bodily parts.

Diagnosis

Because the symptoms of a prostatic abscess might resemble those of other prostate disorders, diagnosing one can be difficult. To confirm the diagnosis, a comprehensive medical history, physical examination, and imaging tests such as an MRI or ultrasound may be required. A sample of the pus may also be taken for laboratory testing to pinpoint the precise bacteria causing the infection.

Treatment Options

Antibiotics are frequently used in conjunction with drainage to treat prostatic abscesses. The specific bacteria that are causing the infection are targeted with antibiotics, which also reduce inflammation. Depending on the size and location of the abscess, drainage may be accomplished via a surgical procedure or a needle aspiration.

A rigorous course of treatment for a prostatic abscess may occasionally necessitate hospitalization. This is particularly true if the illness has migrated to other body areas or if the patient has further underlying medical issues. During hospitalization, the abscess can be treated more forcefully and under strict observation while receiving intravenous antibiotics.

Complications

A prostatic abscess can cause major problems including sepsis, a potentially fatal infection that can spread throughout the body if it is not treated. The prostate gland may also be harmed, which could result in long-term concerns like infertility or urinary issues.

Prevention

Maintaining a healthy prostate and engaging in responsible sexual practice is key to preventing prostatic abscesses. Regular prostate exams and prompt diagnosis and treatment of any prostate infections or disorders can aid in preventing the growth of abscesses. Additionally, the risk of STDs, which can result in prostatic abscesses, can be decreased by using condoms during sexual activity.

Let's sum up by saying that a prostatic abscess is a rare but serious ailment that needs to be treated right away. Complications can be avoided and a full recovery can be encouraged with early diagnosis, treatment with antibiotics, and drainage. The likelihood of getting a prostatic abscess can also be decreased by maintaining good prostate health and engaging in safe sexual practices.

2.5: Prostate Stones

Small mineral deposits that can develop in the prostate gland are referred to as prostate stones or prostatic calculi. Typically innocuous, these stones might not even create any symptoms. Larger stones or a buildup of smaller stones, on the other hand, may cause symptoms like pain during ejaculation, blood in semen, or recurring urinary tract infections.

Prostate-specific antigen (PSA) blood tests and digital rectal exams, which are part of routine prostate exams, are essential for the early identification and treatment of prostate diseases. It is advised to seek medical advice if any alarming symptoms manifest. A qualified healthcare provider can provide a precise diagnosis and recommend the best course of action based on the specific requirements of each patient.

CHAPTER 3: MISCONCEPTIONS ABOUT PROSTATE CONDITION

Myths and false beliefs about prostate health contribute to confusion and misunderstanding.

The following are some widespread misconceptions and beliefs concerning prostate health, along with the facts that dispel them:

Myth: Prostate cancer is always present when a PSA score is high.

Factual statement: Prostate cancer can be detected by a high PSA (prostate-specific antigen) level, but it can also be brought on by other disorders including BPH (benign prostatic hyperplasia) or prostatitis (prostate gland inflammation). Healthcare professionals should assess how to interpret PSA readings to ascertain the source of the spike.

Myth: If a member of your family has prostate cancer, you will too.

Fact: A family history of prostate cancer can raise your risk of getting it, but it doesn't guarantee that you will. Men who have a history of the disease in their families should get regular physicals and may require earlier and more frequent prostate screenings.

Myth: Symptoms of prostate cancer are always present.

Fact: Prostate cancer in its early stages may not show any symptoms. Indicators of advanced growth include frequent urination, difficulty urinating, and a weak urine stream.

Myth: Prostate cancer risk may rise as people age due to family history.

Fact: The prevalence of prostate cancer is higher in males over 50, although it can also strike younger men.

Prostate cancer risk may rise as people age due to family history and other risk factors.

Myth: Prostate massage can treat or prevent prostate cancer.

Fact: There is no proof that prostate massage helps prevent or treat prostate cancer, even though it can help with BPH or prostatitis symptoms. The greatest approaches to identifying prostate cancer early can be done through routine checkups and PSA tests, which can increase the likelihood of effective treatment.

To differentiate fact from fiction regarding prostate health, it is crucial to speak with a healthcare professional. Men may be discouraged from taking proactive steps to maintain prostate health, such as early identification and intervention when necessary, because of misconceptions and myths.

3.1: Frequently asked questions and dispelling of rumors or myths

The following are some often-asked queries and debunkings of myths or falsehoods about prostate health:

Q: Can eating well lower your risk of developing prostate cancer?

A: A balanced diet can help lower the risk of prostate cancer, yes. A diet rich in red and processed meats and saturated fats can increase the risk of prostate cancer, but a diet rich in fruits, vegetables, whole grains, and low-fat dairy can lower it.

Q: Does having a vasectomy put you at a higher risk of prostate cancer?

A: Despite some studies' suggestions to the contrary, the majority of sizable studies have not discovered any appreciable rise in the risk of prostate cancer linked to vasectomy.

Q: The danger of prostate cancer is reduced by frequent ejaculation, right?

A: There is some evidence that regular ejaculation may reduce the incidence of prostate cancer, but further studies are necessary to substantiate this.

Q: Do cyclists have a higher chance of developing prostate cancer?

A: There is currently no proof that cycling raises one's risk of developing prostate cancer. Long periods on a hard or narrow bicycle seat, however, could result in temporary numbness or discomfort.

Q: Should a man with a swollen prostate abstain from having sex?

A: No, guys can still have sex despite having an enlarged prostate. However, some people may have signs like trouble keeping an erection or discomfort when ejaculating during intercourse.

Q: Can herbal remedies treat or prevent prostate cancer?

A: The ability of herbal supplements to prevent or treat prostate cancer remains unproven. Some herbal supplements may be able to reduce the signs and symptoms of an enlarged prostate, but it's crucial to speak with a doctor first before taking any form of supplement.

It's important to keep in mind that, even though myths and rumors may appear to be true, getting the truth is necessary. Men can use this knowledge to make educated decisions to safeguard their well-being and help debunk false beliefs about prostate health.

CHAPTER 4: PROSTATE CANCER

Men's health is significantly affected by prostate cancer, which can be brought on by several factors including age, family history, and ethnicity.

4.1: Factors that Increase the risk of developing prostate cancer

Age

The majority of instances of prostate cancer are found in males over 65, making age a key risk factor for the disease. Men are much more at risk as they age, underscoring the significance of routine testing and education.

Family history

Family history is important because men who had brothers or fathers who have had prostate cancer are more likely to develop the disease themselves. It is advised to begin screenings early and receive more frequent monitoring in such circumstances.

Ethnicity

Prostate cancer risk has been shown to vary by ethnicity, with African-American males seeing the highest incidence rates. Additionally, they are more likely to have their illnesses discovered in their latter stages.

4.2: The different stages of prostate cancer

Both patients and medical professionals must be aware of the various prostate cancer phases. Based on how far it has gone, prostate cancer can be divided into various stages. The patient's suitable treatment options and prospects are determined by this staging. The stages range from early stages where the prostate gland is still the only site of the cancer to advanced stages where it has spread to other distant organs.

Early Stage

The early stages of prostate cancer refer to the initial development and progression of malignant cells within the prostate gland. Understanding these early stages is crucial for early detection and intervention, which significantly improves treatment outcomes and patient survival rates.

Prostate cancer typically begins with the formation of small cancerous cells within the prostate gland. In its early stages, prostate cancer often remains localized, meaning it is confined within the prostate itself and has not spread to other parts of the body. This stage is known as stage I or stage II prostate cancer.

One of the early warning signs of prostate cancer is the presence of elevated levels of prostate-specific antigen (PSA) in the blood. PSA is a protein produced by the prostate gland, and increased levels may indicate the presence of prostate abnormalities, including cancer. However, it's important to note that a high PSA level does not necessarily indicate cancer and may be caused by other non-cancerous conditions as well.

Early-stage prostate cancer usually grows slowly and may not cause noticeable symptoms. However, as the tumor enlarges, it can lead to urinary symptoms such as frequent urination, difficulty starting or stopping urination, weak urinary stream, or blood in the urine. These symptoms may also be associated with benign prostatic hyperplasia (BPH), a non-cancerous condition that causes prostate enlargement.

To diagnose early-stage prostate cancer, doctors may perform a series of tests. This includes a digital rectal examination (DRE), where the physician manually examines the prostate through the rectum to check for any abnormalities or hard nodules. Additionally, a prostate biopsy may be recommended, which involves taking small tissue samples from the prostate to be examined under a microscope for cancerous cells.

Once the diagnosis of early-stage prostate cancer has been established, other examinations including imaging scans (MRI, CT scan, bone scan) may be carried out to ascertain the cancer's extent and whether it has progressed outside of the prostate gland. Cancer staging and therapy choices are guided by this information.

Treatment options for early-stage prostate cancer include active surveillance, surgery, radiation therapy, and hormone therapy. Active surveillance involves closely monitoring the cancer's progression through regular exams and tests, while surgery (prostatectomy) aims to remove the entire prostate gland. Radiation therapy uses high-energy beams to destroy cancer cells, and hormone therapy blocks the production of testosterone (the hormone that fuels prostate cancer growth). The choice of treatment depends on various factors, such as the patient's age, overall health, cancer stage, and personal preferences.

In conclusion, the early stages of prostate cancer involve the initial growth of malignant cells within the prostate gland. Detecting prostate cancer early is crucial for successful treatment outcomes. Regular check-ups, PSA blood tests, and awareness of common symptoms are essential for early detection and prompt intervention. If diagnosed with early-stage prostate cancer, there are several treatment options available, and the choice should be made based on individual circumstances and in consultation with healthcare professionals.

Advanced stage

Prostate cancer is a condition that affects the prostate gland in males, and its progression can be classified into different stages. In the advanced stages of prostate cancer, the disease has spread beyond the prostate and may have affected surrounding tissues or distant areas of the body. Let's explore the characteristics and implications of advanced prostate cancer.

Localized Spread: At this stage, prostate cancer cells may have invaded nearby tissues such as the seminal vesicles, bladder, or rectum. The cancer cells may also have spread to nearby lymph nodes. However, in localized spread, the cancer has not yet reached distant organs.

Regional Spread: Prostate cancer cells can extend further to reach lymph nodes located beyond the vicinity of the prostate gland. Lymph nodes in the pelvic area, such as those near the iliac arteries or retroperitoneal lymph nodes, can be affected. Cancer cells found in regional lymph nodes indicate a more advanced stage of the disease.

Distant Metastasis: In advanced stages, prostate cancer can metastasize or spread to other parts of the body, particularly bone, liver, lungs, or distant lymph nodes. Bones, especially the spine, hips, and pelvis, are the most common sites for prostate cancer metastasis. Metastatic prostate cancer is also associated with a higher risk of developing complications such as fractures or spinal cord compression.

Hormone Resistance: Over time, prostate cancer cells can become resistant to hormone therapy, which is a common treatment approach for this disease. Hormone-resistant prostate cancer, also known as castration-resistant prostate cancer, continues to grow and spread despite hormone therapy, making treatment more challenging.

Symptom Progression: As prostate cancer advances, it can lead to various symptoms. These may include bone pain, especially in the spine, hips, or pelvis, urinary problems such as increased frequency, difficulty urinating, or blood in the urine, erectile dysfunction, weight loss, fatigue, or weakness. Advanced prostate cancer may also cause complications like urinary obstruction or spinal cord compression, which require immediate medical attention.

Treatment options vary depending on the stage and extent of prostate cancer. In advanced stages, treatment approaches commonly include systemic therapies such as chemotherapy, immunotherapy, targeted therapy, or radiopharmaceuticals. These treatments aim to control the spread and growth of cancerous cells and alleviate symptoms. Palliative care, focusing on symptom management and improving the quality of life, is also an essential aspect of advanced prostate cancer management.

Regular monitoring, close communication with healthcare professionals, and adherence to treatment plans are crucial for managing advanced prostate cancer. It's important to note that treatment options and outcomes can vary for each individual, so personalized medical advice from healthcare providers is paramount in developing an effective management strategy.

4.3: Diagnostic procedures

Prostate cancer detection and evaluation depend heavily on diagnostic methods. The prostate-specific antigen (PSA) test, which quantifies levels of a protein created by the prostate gland, is the most widely used screening method. Cancer can be indicated by elevated PSA levels, but additional research is required. This frequently entails a prostate biopsy, in which minute tissue samples are removed from the prostate gland for microscopic analysis.

Depending on the diagnosis and personal health circumstances, there may be a range of therapy choices for prostate issues.

4.4: Treatment options

Depending on the stage and aggressiveness of the cancer, several treatment options are available. For prostate cancer, they may include:

Active surveillance

Also known as watchful waiting, is closely monitoring prostate cancer but delaying the initiation of treatment by routine PSA testing, DREs, and biopsies. Men with low-risk prostate cancer or those with other health issues who would make treatment riskier might benefit from this strategy.

Surgery

Sometimes referred to as radical prostatectomy, removes the prostate gland and the tissues around it. For males with localized prostate cancer, it might be advised. Surgery has the potential to remove malignant tissue, but there are hazards involved, including the possibility of incontinence or impotence.

Radiation therapy

This may be recommended in place of or in addition to surgery. It eliminates cancer cells by employing high-energy rays. It can be used either internally or externally and uses radioactive sources that are put right into the prostate gland.

Hormone therapy

In hormone therapy, male hormones (androgens) that can promote the growth of prostate cancer cells are prevented from being produced. Advanced prostate cancer patients may receive it alone or in conjunction with other treatments.

Chemotherapy

Chemotherapy is a type of systemic medicine that targets and destroys cancer cells all over the body. For males with metastatic or advanced prostate cancer, it might be advised.

In addition to these therapies, a healthcare professional might suggest other measures like:

Cryotherapy is a treatment method that includes briefly subjecting the body to extremely low temperatures. The most typical application is localized therapy. The body is exposed to temperatures below -100 degrees Celsius using a variety of devices, such as ice packs, localized cryotherapy machines, or whole-body cryotherapy chambers.

High-intensity focused ultrasound (HIFU) can be used to treat some tumors in a non-invasive or minimally invasive manner. Compared to conventional surgery or radiation therapy, it has benefits including precision tumor targeting, lesser injury to nearby healthy tissues, and perhaps quicker recovery times.

Or there is immunotherapy, a form of medical care that uses the immune system's power to combat illness, notably cancer. Immunotherapy works by encouraging the body's immune system to recognize and combat cancer cells, in contrast to conventional treatments like chemotherapy and radiation, which directly target the disease.

Numerous forms of cancer have responded remarkably well to immunotherapy, which also has fewer side effects than conventional therapies and the possibility for long-lasting remission. However, it's crucial to remember that not all patients respond to immunotherapy in the same way and that the efficacy can differ based on the type and stage of cancer.

While these treatment options can be effective, they may also come with potential side effects and complications.

4.5: Potential side effects and complications.

Instead of early treatment alternatives like surgery or radiation therapy, active surveillance is a management method utilized in some low-risk prostate cancer cases. It entails routinely tracking cancer with specialized testing to see if the cancer is developing, such as PSA blood tests and prostate biopsies. For qualified applicants, active surveillance is generally regarded as safe and effective, although there are certain potential risks and considerations.

Cancer progression

One of the main worries with active surveillance is the potential for cancer development. Treatment can be required if the cancer begins to advance or spread while the patient is being monitored. Continuous observation is essential to quickly spot any signs of development.

Anxiety and psychological effects

For some people, having an untreated cancer diagnosis can result in anxiety and psychological anguish. Cancer patients and their families may experience emotional distress as a result of their ongoing awareness of the disease and the uncertainty surrounding its course.

Delayed treatment

Delaying decisive treatment while under active surveillance. This delay may prevent some patients from taking advantage of more suitable therapy options. Treatment outcomes could suffer if cancer dramatically advances while being monitored.

Active surveillance necessitates recurrent invasive follow-up examinations, such as repeat biopsies. Risks associated with these treatments include those related to pain, bleeding, infection, and anesthesia-related problems.

Impact on quality of life

Prostate cancer treatment may have an impact on aspects like bowel habits, sexual function, and urine function. Active surveillance, on the other hand, seeks to reduce the impact on quality of life by postponing action unless essential. However, if further treatment is required, the possibility of treatment-related side effects still exists.

Patient compliance is essential for regular monitoring, which is a requirement of active surveillance. To ensure that the cancer is adequately monitored, regular follow-up visits, exams, and appointments are required. Failure to follow monitoring protocols may cause progression indicators to be overlooked.

It is crucial to remember that choosing to pursue active monitoring should be done in cooperation with medical experts who can evaluate the individual's particular circumstance and offer tailored advice. Throughout the active surveillance period, regular and open communication with the medical team is crucial to address any concerns, monitor changes, and guarantee appropriate management.

Surgery-related problems

Prostate surgery-related complications can take several different forms.

Urine incontinence

Following prostate surgery, some patients may have urine incontinence that may be temporary or permanent and manifest as anything from little leakage to total loss of bladder control. This happens as a result of the surgery harming the nerves or urinary sphincter.

Erectile dysfunction

Prostate surgery, including radical prostatectomy, may cause erectile dysfunction. This occurs as a result of the surgery's damage to or removal of the nerves and blood arteries necessary for achieving and sustaining an erection.

Urinary retention

Surgical operations occasionally result in urinary retention, which is when the bladder cannot be completely emptied and requires the use of a catheter to drain the urine.

Infection

There is a danger of infection following surgery. Urinary tract infections, wound infections, or even life-threatening infections like sepsis, may occur after prostate surgery. These infections need to be treated by a doctor right away.

Blood loss

There is a chance of considerable blood loss after prostate surgery. Although precautions are taken to reduce this danger, Blood transfusions or extra surgical intervention may be necessary to manage excessive bleeding.

Bladder neck contracture

In some instances, the bladder neck can develop scar tissue, which results in a condition known as bladder neck contracture. Urination may become tough as a result, which may call for additional assistance to fix.

Bowel issues

Some people could develop bowel issues after prostate surgery. This may involve problems including diarrhea, intestinal urgency, or constipation. Although they often get better with time, some issues may call for medication or dietary changes.

Fecal incontinence, which is the inability to control bowel motions, can occur as an uncommon side effect of surgery. This problem can be difficult to manage and may need expert care.

It is crucial to remember that not everyone will have these side effects, and the probability can change based on the precise surgical approach employed, the patient's general health, and the surgeon's level of skill. Before undertaking the surgical operation, it is crucial to have a full talk with your healthcare physician to understand the potential risks and advantages.

Prostate cancer is frequently treated with radiation therapy, but like any medical procedure, it has possible dangers and side effects. The following are a few risks connected to prostate radiation therapy:

Fatigue

One of radiation therapy's most frequent adverse effects is fatigue. Patients may feel generally worn out and uninspired when inside the tent. This may have an impact on everyday activities and call for more rest.

Radiation therapy for the prostate may result in urinary issues such as increased frequency, urgency, or trouble urinating. Urinary incontinence, which can be either temporary or permanent depending on the patient, may also occur in some patients.

Bowel issues

Radiation can also have an impact on the rectum and result in bowel issues. This could involve intestinal urgency, rectal bleeding, or diarrhea. Though they frequently get better with time, these symptoms sometimes linger.

Sexual dysfunction

Radiation therapy may cause problems with erections or diminished libido. Depending on a person's unique circumstances and previous sexual function, the severity of these issues may vary.

Skin reactions

Radiation exposure can cause the skin in the treatment region to become sensitive, irritated, or red. This may result in irritation, itching, and occasionally skin peeling.

Long-term side effects

Some patients may experience long-term side effects that appear months or even years after radiation treatment. These can include ongoing bowel or bladder issues, as well as secondary cancers in rare circumstances.

It's crucial to remember that not every patient will suffer from these issues and that each person will experience side effects differently. To control and reduce these risks, healthcare professionals collaborate closely with patients. If it's necessary to address certain issues and enhance the quality of life while and after treatment, they may provide supportive care techniques, drugs, or referrals to experts.

Prostate cancer patients frequently choose hormone therapy, also known as androgen deprivation therapy (ADT). Although it has the potential to halt the development and spread of cancer cells, it is not without risk. The following are some risks connected with using hormone therapy to treat prostate cancer:

Hormone therapy can have a severe negative impact on a man's sexual function. It might result in erectile dysfunction, lowered libido (sex drive), and trouble getting or keeping an erection. These adverse effects may deteriorate a patient's quality of life and last long after hormone therapy is stopped.

Hot flashes

A typical adverse effect of hormone therapy is hot flashes, which are comparable to menopausal women's symptoms. They are distinguished by abrupt sensations of heat, which are frequently accompanied by perspiration and flushing. Even while hot flashes are typically transient, they can be uncomfortable and interfere with regular tasks.

Osteoporosis and bone thinning

Hormone therapy may result in a loss of bone density, increasing the risk of fractures. For older men who may already be at risk for osteoporosis, this is especially troubling. To reduce this risk, regular bone density testing and the proper dietary supplements or medications may be required.

Fatigue and energy loss

Many men receiving hormone therapy report feeling tired and lacking in energy. This may affect daily functioning and can be ascribed to hormonal changes. This side effect can be reduced by getting enough sleep and controlling your stress levels.

Mood swings, anger, and depression can all be attributed to hormonal variations brought on by hormone therapy. Any changes in mood or emotional well-being should be discussed by patients with their healthcare team, as appropriate interventions, including counseling or medication, may be suggested.

Hormone therapy has the potential to cause metabolic abnormalities, such as weight gain, elevated cholesterol levels, and a higher risk of developing diabetes. The risks can be reduced by eating a balanced diet, exercising frequently, and keeping an eye on certain metabolic indicators.

Cardiovascular complications

Some research raises the possibility that hormone therapy may increase the risk of cardiovascular issues like heart disease and stroke. Pre-existing cardiovascular problems should be closely evaluated and treated appropriately in patients.

It's crucial to remember that not all individuals will experience these adverse effects and that each person may experience side effects differently in terms of severity and length. Before beginning hormone therapy, the medical team should go over these potential side effects with the patient. They should also keep a line of communication open throughout the treatment to address any issues that may come up.

Advanced prostate cancer is frequently treated with chemotherapy. Although it has the potential to reduce tumor size and limit the spread of the disease, it is also linked to several negative side effects. The following are some typical issues that can develop while using chemotherapy for prostate cancer:

weariness

Chemotherapy's side effects include excessive weariness. This may be because chemotherapy medications also harm healthy cells, which results in general weakness and a lack of energy.

Nausea and vomiting

A lot of chemotherapy medications can make you feel queasy and sick. Anti-nausea drugs are frequently used to manage these adverse effects, while they might not completely get rid of them.

Hair loss

One well-known adverse effect of many chemotherapy treatments is hair loss, often known as alopecia. Loss of hair on the scalp as well as hair on other body parts, like the eyebrows and eyelashes, can be a result of this.

Weakening of the immune system

Chemotherapy can impair immunity, rendering a patient more prone to infections and diseases. This is because the medications may have an impact on the development of white blood cells, which are essential for warding off infections.

Increased risk of bleeding and bruising

Certain chemotherapy medications may impair the body's capacity to form blood clots, which increases the risk of bleeding and bruising. Chemotherapy sufferers must keep a tight eye out for any bleeding or bruising and report it to their medical team.

Peripheral neuropathy

Chemotherapy medications can harm peripheral nerves, resulting in symptoms including tingling, numbness, or pain in the hands and feet.

Bowel and bladder issues

Chemotherapy might result in gastrointestinal symptoms like constipation or diarrhea. Additionally, some patients may have urine incontinence or irritation of the bladder.

Weight changes

Some people may gain or lose weight while receiving chemotherapy. This may be caused by several things, including adjustments in appetite, metabolism, or fluid retention.

It is important to remember that not every patient will suffer from these side effects, and their severity might vary based on personal traits and the particular chemotherapy regimen used. To manage and address any issues that may emerge during chemotherapy treatment, patients must regularly communicate with their healthcare team.

It is expedient to go over all of your treatment options with your doctor and assess the benefits and drawbacks of each. Age, general health, and personal preferences can all have an impact on treatment choices.

The fact that every person's experience with prostate cancer and its treatment will be unique should also be mentioned. Patients and their families must get continual support and guidance from healthcare experts as they travel through this difficult journey.

CHAPTER 5: BENIGN PROSTATIC HYPERPLASIA (BPH)

A benign prostate gland growth is known as benign prostatic hyperplasia (BPH). The prostate is a walnut-sized gland that is situated below the bladder and next to the urethra, the tube that is in charge of removing pee from the body. Urinary issues may result from the pressure the enlarged prostate puts on the urethra.

5.1: Its impact on urinary function

Depending on the degree of prostate enlargement, BPH can have a modest to severe effect on urine function.

Increased frequency of urine, a weak urinary stream, difficulties initiating and halting urination, incomplete bladder emptying, and urinary urgency are typical symptoms.

BPH can cause renal issues, bladder stones, infections, and urine retention in more severe situations.

5.2: How it is diagnosed

A doctor will often study the patient's medical history, perform a physical exam, and run many tests to determine whether the patient has BPH. A digital rectal exam to evaluate the size and health of the prostate, a urine test to rule out infections, a blood test to evaluate kidney function, and perhaps imaging tests like an ultrasound or cystoscopy are among these.

5.3: Treatment options

Various strategies can be used to control BPH, depending on the extent of the symptoms, how they affect a patient's quality of life, and other factors specific to that patient.

From conservative methods to surgical techniques, there are several different BPH treatment options.

The first line of treatment for mild to moderate BPH symptoms is frequent medication. Drugs like alpha-blockers and 5-alpha reductase inhibitors are frequently recommended. The prostate and bladder neck muscles are relaxed by alpha-blockers, which improves urine flow. On the other hand, 5-alpha reductase inhibitors shrink the prostate by obstructing the hormones that encourage its growth.

Another alternative for treating BPH is less invasive methods. These techniques try to treat urinary problems without using open surgery. Examples include laser therapies, transurethral needle ablation, and transurethral microwave thermotherapy. These treatments, which can be done as an outpatient, often use heat or laser radiation to shrink the prostate and increase urine flow.

Surgery may be advised in circumstances where drugs and less invasive techniques are inadequate or prostate enlargement is significant. A popular surgical treatment called transurethral resection of the prostate (TURP) involves removing extra prostate tissue through the urethra. Other surgical procedures include open prostate surgery, such as a straightforward prostatectomy, and laser prostatectomy.

The intensity of the symptoms, the size of the prostate, the patient's general health, and personal preferences all play a role in the treatment decision. It's crucial to have a lengthy conversation with a medical expert to decide on the best course of action for treating BPH in each case.

CHAPTER 6: PROSTATITIS

Inflammation of the prostate gland, which is a tiny, walnut-shaped gland found under the bladder in males, is the hallmark of the disorder known as prostatitis.

6.1: Types of prostatitis

Acute bacterial prostatitis, chronic bacterial prostatitis, nonbacterial prostatitis, and asymptomatic inflammatory prostatitis are a few of the several forms of prostatitis.

Acute bacterial prostatitis

This kind of prostatitis is brought on by a bacterial infection and is frequently characterized by the abrupt development of symptoms including intense pain in the lower abdomen, pelvis, or lower back, frequent urination urges, trouble urinating, fever, and chills.

A physical examination, medical history, urine culture, and occasionally a prostate fluid culture is used to make the diagnosis.

Antibiotics, painkillers, and plenty of fluids are frequently used as treatments. Severe instances may necessitate hospitalization.

Recurrent urinary tract infections brought on by the presence of bacteria in the prostate gland characterize chronic bacterial prostatitis.

Pelvic pain, frequent urination, painful urination, and discomfort after ejaculation are possible symptoms.

A complete medical history, physical examination, cultures of the urine and prostate fluid, and maybe imaging tests are all required for the diagnosis.

Long-term antibiotic therapy, painkillers, and lifestyle changes may all be used as treatment options.

Nonbacterial prostatitis

This type of prostatitis, which is the most prevalent, develops when there is inflammation of the prostate but no apparent bacterial infection. Although the precise etiology is unknown, it might be related to prior infections, abnormalities in the pelvic floor muscles, or autoimmune conditions.

Pelvic pain, vaginal discomfort, frequent urination, and pain during ejaculation are a few symptoms that may be present.

The diagnosis is made after ruling out a bacterial infection and considering the symptoms.

Through pain treatment, dietary changes (such as abstaining from coffee and alcohol), physical therapy, and relaxation methods, symptoms are treated.

Asymptomatic inflammatory prostatitis

Although there are no obvious symptoms in this form of prostatitis, inflammation can be seen when checking for other illnesses.

Treatment might not be required until symptoms appear.

The management of prostatitis might include lifestyle changes in addition to the use of antibiotics and painkillers.

A lifestyle change may involve avoiding irritants like caffeine and spicy foods, consuming more fluids, maintaining good cleanliness, engaging in regular exercise, learning stress management skills, and performing pelvic floor exercises.

A healthcare specialist should be consulted to identify the precise type of prostatitis and create a customized treatment plan.

CHAPTER 7: LIFESTYLE HABITS THAT CAN REDUCE THE RISK OF PROSTATE PROBLEMS

To support prostate health and lower the risk of prostate issues, a healthy lifestyle must be maintained.

Following are some dietary suggestions and ways of living that can be beneficial:

Balanced Diet

A healthy diet is essential for promoting prostate health. The necessary vitamins, minerals, and antioxidants found in a range of fruits and vegetables can assist your body in fighting prostate issues. Daily fruit and vegetable consumption should be at least five servings.

Products Made From Tomatoes

Because tomato-based foods include a lot of lycopene, a potent antioxidant, including them in your diet may be advantageous. Lycopene may help lower the likelihood of prostate issues, according to studies. Include cooked tomatoes, tomato paste, or tomato sauce in your meals.

Healthy Fats

Choose unsaturated fats like those in nuts, seeds, fatty fish (like salmon and tuna), and olive oil. Omega-3 fatty acids, which are included in these fats and have anti-inflammatory characteristics, may support prostate health.

Reduce the amount of processed meals and red meat you consume. It's best to moderate how much of these things you eat. An elevated risk of prostate issues has been linked to a high intake of these foods. Instead, choose lean protein sources like tofu, fish, poultry, and lentils.

Remain Hydrated

Water consumption is crucial for maintaining overall health, including prostate health. To aid in the body's ability to rid itself of toxins, aim for at least 8 glasses of water each day.

Frequent Exercise

Maintaining a healthy weight and lowering the risk of prostate issues require frequent physical activity. Aim for 150 minutes or more per week of moderate-intensity aerobic exercise, such as brisk walking or cycling.

Maintain a Healthy Weight

Prostate issues are more likely to develop in those who are overweight or obese. Put your attention on maintaining a healthy weight by engaging in regular exercise and eating a balanced diet.

Limit your intake of alcohol and coffee because both substances might make prostate issues worse. Aim to restrict your coffee intake and drink alcohol in moderation.

Avoid Smoking

Smoking has been associated with a higher incidence of prostate issues. Quitting smoking is good for your general health as well as your prostate health.

Maintaining proper hygiene can help prevent urinary tract infections and other disorders that could harm the prostate gland, even if it may not have a direct impact on prostate health.

Regular Medical Check-ups

Regular prostate screenings are essential for early detection of any abnormalities or potential issues. Consult with your healthcare provider to determine the appropriate age and frequency for prostate-specific antigen (PSA) tests and other screenings.

Stress Management

Chronic stress can weaken the immune system and negatively impact prostate health. Engage in stress-reducing activities such as mindfulness, meditation, yoga, or hobbies that help relax the mind and body.

Adequate Restful Sleep

Getting enough quality sleep is vital for overall health and well-being, including prostate health. Each night, try to get 7-8 hours of unbroken sleep.

Prostate-Supportive Supplements

Some natural supplements like saw palmetto, beta-sitosterol, and lycopene have been associated with supporting prostate health. Before introducing any supplements into your routine, you should speak with a healthcare provider.

It's crucial to keep in mind that living a healthy lifestyle is only one factor in prostate health. For the early discovery and management of any potential prostate issues, routine medical examinations and screenings are also essential.

CHAPTER 8: SCREENING AND PREVENTION

Regular screening is crucial since prostate cancer is frequently slow-growing and may not exhibit any signs in its early stages. The two most popular procedures for finding prostate cancer early are:

The PSA blood test or prostate-specific antigen

Digital rectal examination (DRE).

8.1: The PSA blood test or Prostate-specific antigen

The PSA test quantifies the blood's concentration of PSA protein. A high PSA level can be a sign of prostate cancer, but it can also be brought on by other issues with the prostate, like BPH. Despite being widely used, the

PSA test has come under fire for providing false positive results that might prompt unneeded biopsies and treatment.

8.2: Digital Rectal Examination

To feel the prostate gland, a healthcare professional performs a physical examination known as a "digital rectal exam" (DRE). Although this examination might be painful, it is a quick and efficient way to find any variations in the prostate gland's shape or texture.

Additional testing may be advised if a PSA or DRE results in an anomaly. A prostate biopsy, in which small tissue samples are obtained from the prostate gland and examined for cancer cells, may be part of this process. Prostate cancer and other prostate issues may also be diagnosed with the aid of imaging tests like an MRI or an ultrasound.

8.3: Weighing the pros and cons of PSA testing

Prostate-specific antigen (PSA) testing is one method of prostate cancer screening that continues to spark debate in the medical profession. Prostate cancer screening seeks to find the disease when it's still treatable. However, it is important to carefully weigh the advantages and disadvantages of PSA testing.

One benefit of PSA testing is that it can identify prostate cancer in its early stages, which raises the possibility of effective treatment. People who desire to take control of their health may find peace of mind from it as well. Furthermore, PSA testing enables people who are at higher risk to be identified, such as those with a family history of prostate cancer, so that proper preventive actions can be taken.

PSA testing, on the other hand, has several drawbacks. The test is non-specific for prostate cancer and has the potential to produce false positives, which can cause unwarranted worry, invasive follow-up treatments, and possible overtreatment. In other circumstances, therapy for prostate cancer may not be essential because it can be slow-growing and may not present any symptoms or harm over a person's lifespan. When it comes to PSA testing, there are worries about overdiagnosis and overtreatment.

Based on thorough research and data, respected groups have created guidelines to address this controversy. For instance, the United States Preventive Services Task Force (USPSTF) advises people and healthcare practitioners to collaborate when making decisions about PSA testing. They recommend that males aged 55 to 69 have a one-on-one conversation about the advantages and hazards before making an informed decision.

8.4: Regular check-ups

There are other preventive steps that people should be aware of in addition to PSA testing. The importance of routine examinations and prostate health conversations with a medical expert cannot be overstated. Knowing one's family history might also aid in identifying those who are more vulnerable. People may need to start screening sooner or be more cautious in monitoring their prostate health if there is a family history of the disease.

Furthermore, it's crucial to be aware of early warning indicators and symptoms. These symptoms could include erectile dysfunction, inability to urinate, frequent urination (particularly at night), blood in the urine or semen, pelvic pain, or frequent urination. It is advised to seek immediate medical advice if any of these symptoms are present.

Making informed judgments is crucial, as the heated topic of prostate cancer screening highlights. Although PSA testing may aid in the early detection of prostate cancer, it also has risks like false positive readings and possibly overtreatment. Adhering to guidelines issued by reputable organizations, taking part in shared decision-making with medical professionals, being proactive about arranging routine check-ups, and being aware of one's family history are all ways that individuals can make informed decisions about their prostate health.

CHAPTER 9: EMOTIONAL AND PSYCHOLOGICAL CONSIDERATIONS

The general health of people with prostate-related disorders is significantly influenced by emotional and psychological factors.

The possible emotional effects that these illnesses may have on men and their relationships must be acknowledged and addressed. Here are some important things to think about:

Recognize your feelings

Receiving a prostate-related diagnosis may cause you to experience a variety of emotions, such as fear, anxiety, grief, and anger. Instead of repressing these emotions, it's critical to allow yourself to feel and express them. Discuss your feelings with your doctor, friends, or loved ones.

Ask for help

It's important to establish a strong support system. Make contact with organizations, online communities, or counseling services that focus on prostate-related issues. These platforms give people the chance to connect with others who are experiencing similar things, exchange experiences and insights, and get help. Be in the company of understanding and encouraging people who can boost your emotional well-being.

Express yourself honestly

It's important to express yourself honestly to your partner. Share your thoughts and worries about your prostate-related issue. Engage your partner in the decision-making process because their understanding and support can improve your mental health.

Upgrade your knowledge about your ailment and available therapies. You can reduce uncertainty and gain the ability to make well-informed decisions by having a thorough understanding of the condition and its treatment. For accurate and current information, check out dependable resources including trusted medical books, websites, and healthcare specialists.

Practice self-care

Look after your mental health by taking part in relaxing and stress-relieving activities. This could be doing regular exercise, practicing meditation, doing deep breathing exercises, engaging in hobbies, or doing things that make you happy and fulfilled. Put self-care first to keep a good outlook during diagnosis, treatment, and survival.

Ask for professional assistance if necessary

If you discover that your emotional health has been seriously impacted, think about getting in touch with a therapist or counselor who has experience with prostate-related disorders. They can offer direction, coping mechanisms, and methods to deal with the emotional difficulties brought on by your diagnosis.

Keep in mind that mental health is a crucial component of total wellness. You may manage this road with resiliency and keep a happy attitude in life by acknowledging the potential emotional burden of prostate-related diseases, getting assistance, and using coping mechanisms.

9.1: Interviews with men who have dealt with prostate problems

1. Arthur, 60: Survivor of prostate cancer

What were your main worries after learning you had prostate cancer?

A: Not knowing what to anticipate and wondering about the future were my two major worries. The potential negative effects of the treatment also caused me a great deal of anxiety.

Describe your symptoms.

A: My diagnosis caught me off guard because I had no symptoms. My cancer was only discovered after a normal physical examination.

What examinations and procedures did you have?

A: A prostate biopsy confirmed that I had cancer. My doctor and I discussed our options and agreed on a radiation therapy regimen.

What suggestions would you make to other men dealing with prostate cancer?

A: I would advise other men to stay knowledgeable and educated about their illnesses, discuss all of their alternatives with their doctor, and maintain a positive outlook.

2. Austin, 45: Benign prostate enlargement

What worries did you have after learning that you had benign prostate enlargement?

A: The persistent urge to urinate was my major worry. It was making my daily routine difficult and uncomfortable.

Describe your symptoms.

A: I was having frequent urination, trouble starting to urinate, a weak stream, and the sensation that my bladder wasn't empty enough.

What examinations and procedures did you have?

A digital rectal exam (DRE), a urinary flow test, and a prostate-specific antigen (PSA) test were all advised by my doctor. I was given medicine to help reduce my prostate based on the test results.

What suggestions do you have for other men dealing with benign prostate enlargement?

A frequent exam with your doctor can help you keep on top of your prostate health, and I would advise other guys to do the same. Never hesitate to bring up any changes in your urinary symptoms, and always heed your doctor's advice regarding screens and treatments.

9.2: Inspiring stories of men who have successfully maintained their prostate health

1. David, 50: Diet and exercise help prevent prostate cancer.

David was worried about his own risk because prostate cancer ran in his family. He began to pay attention to his diet, increasing the amount of fruits, vegetables, and whole grains he consumed while decreasing the amount of red meat and processed meals. He began a daily fitness regimen that included walking, jogging, and strength training in addition to adopting a healthier diet.

His doctor discovered increased PSA levels at his annual exam and advised a prostate biopsy. Although the results of the biopsy were negative, David persisted in maintaining his diet and exercise regimen. His PSA levels stabilized six months later.

David encourages other men to adopt a similar way of life by attributing his proactive attitude to his prostate health through nutrition and exercise to promote his overall health and well-being.

2. Tom, 65: Early detection is the key to treating prostate cancer.

Tom got a standard PSA test, and the results were elevated. He was identified as having prostate cancer following a biopsy. He decided to have a minimally invasive procedure called a robot-assisted laparoscopic prostatectomy, which included removing the prostate gland.

Tom was cancer-free and able to lead an active lifestyle after surgery and a few weeks of rehabilitation. He now serves as an ambassador for prostate cancer early diagnosis and proactive treatment, informing other men about the value of routine checkups and screenings.

3. Mark, 55: Using medicine and lifestyle modifications to treat benign prostate enlargement

For several months, Mark had been dealing with the symptoms of benign prostate enlargement, which were interfering with his regular activities. His issue was identified when he discussed his symptoms with his doctor.

In addition to changing his lifestyle to maintain the health of his prostate, Mark took the medicine the doctor suggested to assist in reducing his prostate. He cut back on alcohol consumption, gave up smoking, and started working out frequently.

Mark's symptoms were much reduced by medication and lifestyle modifications, and he was able to return to his regular activities pain-free. He now leads a healthy, active lifestyle and inspires other guys to take charge of their prostate health.

4. John, 58: Coping with the news that he has prostate cancer

It's terrifying to hear the term "prostate cancer". Upon learning of the diagnosis, I was struck with anxiety and trepidation about what lay ahead. How am I going to get through this, I kept thinking. What sort of medical treatment should I receive? Will my quality of life decline?

However, I managed to maintain my optimism with the help of my loving family, a reliable medical staff, and my faith. I discovered that talking to your doctor and asking questions are two of the most crucial things to do when managing prostate cancer. Making educated choices required knowledge of my diagnosis and my available treatment options.

Years after being diagnosed, my cancer has been effectively treated, and I still get checkups regularly. I now enjoy every day to the fullest and treasure every second spent with my loved ones.

5. Ben, 63: Managing the signs of benign prostatic hyperplasia (BPH)

"It was annoying and difficult when I first started to develop BPH symptoms. I had to get up several times during the night to use the restroom, and even during the day, I felt the need to go frequently.

But I didn't want to accept these symptoms as my lot in life. I spoke with my doctor, who gave me some pharmaceutical recommendations and made some simple lifestyle recommendations that would help with my problems. Reducing coffee and alcohol intake as well as making sure to get enough water were part of this.

I was able to successfully manage my BPH symptoms with the help of my doctor, and as a result, my quality of life greatly increased. Since incorporating these healthy routines into my life, I feel generally better and more energized".

6. Greg, 62: A good diet and regular exercise can help prevent prostate issues.

"I take care to take a preventative approach to my health because I have a family history of prostate issues. I maintain a healthy lifestyle that includes frequent exercise, a balanced diet of whole foods, and regular visits with my primary care physician.

I feel more in charge of my health and less concerned about any future prostate issues as a result. Additionally, I feel better physically and have more energy for my everyday tasks.

I believe that it is worthwhile to put in the work required to maintain a healthy lifestyle. I am aware that by making these minor changes, I am lowering my chance of prostate issues and raising my general standard of living.

These tales emphasize the value of proactive prostate health care, which includes good lifestyle choices, early identification, and efficient treatments.

CHAPTER 10: ADVANCES AND FUTURE DIRECTIONS

Certainly! Prostate health research has made great progress, with several new developments in diagnostic methods, therapeutic modalities, and continuing clinical trials. The diagnosis and treatment of prostate diseases may be improved as a result of these discoveries. The following are some important highlights:

Diagnostic Methods

The diagnosis of prostate cancer has been transformed by the development of cutting-edge imaging tools like multiparametric magnetic resonance imaging (mpMRI). By combining various imaging sequences, mpMRI creates detailed images of the prostate that enable doctors to precisely pinpoint worrisome spots for targeted biopsies. Additionally, non-invasive alternatives to conventional tissue biopsies, such as liquid biopsies and biomarker testing, are being developed to find genetic alterations connected to prostate cancer as well as circulating tumor cells in blood samples.

Precision Medicine

The use of precision medicine techniques is becoming more popular in the management of prostate cancer. Tumor genetic and molecular profiling provides individualized treatment plans and targeted medicines based on the unique tumor characteristics of each patient. This strategy shows potential for better treatment results and fewer adverse effects.

Immunotherapy

This innovative field of study tries to use the immune system of the body to combat prostate cancer. Clinical trials are demonstrating the potential of approaches like immune checkpoint inhibitors and therapeutic cancer vaccines, opening up new treatment options for advanced prostate cancer.

Targeted medicines

To address particular molecular abnormalities in prostate cancer cells, novel targeted medicines are being developed. For instance, in patients with advanced prostate cancer who have grown resistant to traditional hormone therapy, specific inhibitors of the androgen receptor pathway, such as enzalutamide and abiraterone, have demonstrated notable success.

Clinical Studies in Progress

Several clinical studies are currently being conducted to examine emerging technologies, find novel therapy combinations, and assess new treatment alternatives. These studies seek to enhance patient quality of life, lessen side effects, and improve treatment outcomes.

Although these developments appear promising, it's crucial to keep in mind that they are still in various phases of development and might not apply to everyone. To learn about the best diagnostic and treatment options based on their unique requirements and circumstances, people need to speak with healthcare specialists.

CONCLUSION

The ground-breaking book "Prostate Health Revolution: Empowering Men to Take Control of Their Well-Being" clarifies the significance of prostate health and encourages men to take control of their well-being. The numerous facets of prostate health, such as typical conditions, risk factors, preventative tactics, and treatment alternatives, have been covered throughout the book.

The importance of early detection and routine screenings is one of the main lessons to be learned from this book. This book attempts to lessen the stigma around prostate health and promote open dialogues about this crucial part of men's well-being by stressing the significance of routine check-ups and urging men to be proactive about their health.

Additionally, "Prostate Health Revolution" offers insightful information on lifestyle modifications that can dramatically enhance prostate health. This book provides a thorough approach to enhancing prostate health, covering everything from dietary adjustments to exercise regimens, and stress management techniques to the use of natural supplements.

One of the most important lessons to take away from this book is the value of routine testing and early detection. By highlighting the significance of routine check-ups and challenging men to be proactive about their health, this book seeks to reduce the stigma surrounding prostate health and foster open talks about this important aspect of men's well-being.

Additionally, "Prostate Health Revolution" explores the most recent developments in medical technology and prostate issue treatment choices. This book gives men the information they need to make wise health decisions, from conventional procedures to cutting-edge ones.

In the end, "Prostate Health Revolution: Empowering Men to Take Control of Their Well-Being" offers a thorough resource that equips men to give their prostate health priority. This book intends to create a revolution in men's health, where people take active measures to improve their well-being, by offering helpful information, useful advice, and inspirational anecdotes.

We hope that readers will feel empowered as we wrap up this book to take charge of their prostate health, have open discussions about it, and make decisions that will improve their general well-being. Remember, you are in control of your health, and by adopting the ideas presented in this book, you can start living a better, happier life.

www.ingramcontent.com/pod-product-compliance
Lightning Source LLC
Chambersburg PA
CBHW070838260726
48660CB00005B/2080